Vital Bites: An Anthology of Healthful Snacking for Discerning Adults

Stephen N. Arnold

Contents

The Importance of Healthy Snacking

Consuming nutritious snacks regularly is essential to achieving and sustaining a high level of well-being and has many other positive effects. Snacks are frequently considered to be supplementary foods to our regular meals. Yet, they require additional consideration due to their capacity to nourish and maintain energy levels throughout the day. This discussion explains the logic behind including snacks in a healthy diet. It outlines the numerous benefits of making informed decisions regarding the foods you consume between meals. To begin, it is essential to acknowledge the role that snacking might play in maintaining stable glucose levels. When meals are consumed on a conventional three-hour-a-day schedule without any underlying sources of nutrition, it is not unusual for abrupt spikes and blood sugar declines.

Snacking deliberately, on the other hand, can help prevent these swings by ensuring a consistent supply of energy and, as a result, preventing the feelings of loneliness that frequently accompany a sharp decline in glucose levels. In addition, regulating one's appetite can be made more accessible by adding nutrient-dense snacks to one's regular eating routine. When individuals consume smaller, more nutritious snacks that quench hunger between meals, there is less chance that they will eat during their primary meals. This can also assist in maintaining a healthy weight or contribute to efforts to lose weight by limiting eating due to excess hunger, a common cause of weight gain. A further important consideration to consider is that snacks provide an additional chance to consume nutrients, which may or may not be delivered in suitable quantities by main meals. For instance, fulfilling the daily guidelines for vitamins, minerals, and other essential nutrients by snacking on various fruits, vegetables, nuts, and seeds will assist. These foods can be consumed in the form of a variety of foods. The effect of eating nutritious snacks on one's mental function is equally significant. Snacks that are high in nutrients can improve cognitive function, concentration, and memory recall. This is especially true for snacks rich in protein and fat and specific vitamins and minerals known to assist healthy brain function.

Snacks can also play an essential role in providing energy for those who engage in regular physical activity because they can help with exercise and recreation. Snacks eaten at the right time and with the right food can improve athletic performance and make it easier for people to recover after a workout. Children and teenagers, who must consume sufficient nutrients to grow and mature, stand to gain a great deal from developing good snacking habits. Schools have recognized the significance of this, so policies that encourage the consumption of nutritious snacks have been implemented. Overall, it is essential to differentiate between snacks that are good for one's health and those that could harm one's health. The consumption of highly processed snacks, which are frequently loaded with added sugars, salts, and bad fats, must be avoided in favor of consuming foods that have not been subjected to any processing. As this discussion has demonstrated conclusively, an individual's general health and sense of well-being can be significantly impacted by the choice of snacks they consume and the timing of those snacks. It is in our best interest to carefully consider our snacks and be aware of the advantages of including nutritious snacks in our daily routine.

Understanding Nutritional Requirements

An investigation into dietary requirements must consider both macronutrients and micronutrients, which are fundamental to maintaining human health. A thousand words long, this discussion will highlight the importance of eating a balanced diet and the consequences of not getting enough of certain nutrients. The human body requires nourishment, not just nutrition; it involves divided food, including carbs, proteins, fats, vitamins, minerals, and water. Each performs a one-of-a-kind function. The primary source of energy for the body is carbohydrates. Proteins, made up of amino acids, are essential for the growth and repair of tissues. Lipids, most often known as fats, are essential components of cellular structure and are responsible for energy storage. Even though they are not digested, the dietary fibers are crucial for keeping our bodies healthy. Vitamins and minerals, despite being needed in tiny amounts, are necessary to operate all metabolic pathways in the body effectively. The importance of water to the functioning of all life processes is frequently undeniable. Larger quantities of macronutrients are required for optimal health. Consuming carbohydrates from complex sources, such as whole grains, is recommended for optimal health. Proteins are essential for various cellular processes, from enzymatic reactions to supporting structural components. Saturated and unsaturated lipids must be appropriately proportioned to keep one's health in check. A wide variety of vitamins and minerals are included in the category of micronutrients.

Along with the B-complement vitamins, vitamins A, C, D, E, and K are necessary for the production of energy, the function of the immune system, the coagulation of blood, and other cellular processes. Calcium, potassium, and iron are examples of minerals that are crucially important for the transmission of neural signals, the contraction of muscles, and the delivery of oxygen, respectively. Consuming various foods to satisfy the body's requirements for each nutrient is essential to achieving adequate nutrition. This is more important than simply consuming enough calories. UN can both be symptoms of the condition known as malnutrition. Both ends of the range pose severe dangers to public health. Inadequate nutrition can result in illnesses such as anemia, caused by a lack of iron, or scurvy, caused by a lack of vitamin C. The combination of an excessive caloric intake and a lack of proper physical exercise can lead to obesity, which in turn can induce obesity, cardiovascular illnesses, and type 2 debates. It is essential to be aware that different people have different requirements. Age, gender, activity level, and the prevalence of any undeniable health issues are all factors. Folic acid consumption should be increased during pregnancy, for instance, to reduce the risk of chronic birth defects. Athletes might require more protein than average to maintain and develop their muscles. On food labels, recommended dietary allowances (draws) or daily values (doves) are the techniques most typically used to refer to daily nutritional requirements. These recommendations offer guidelines for the average daily consumption amount that should be sufficient to meet the dietary needs of most adults in good health. The choices that you make for your diet ought to strive for variety, equilibrium, and moderation. Most dietary requirements can be met by consuming a diet abundant in fruits, vegetables, lean proteins, whole grains, and healthy fats. Although there are circumstances in which substitution might be advantageous, it should never be used in place of a balanced and divided diet.

Smart Snacking Strategies

Developing a compendium on "Smart Snacking Strategies" calls for a discussion on the science of nutrition and the practices of individual consumers. One shall make an effort, within the confines of a word count of one thousand, to provide a page of utility and cognizance to individuals looking to navigate the complicated terrain of healthy eating. Conscious Approaches to Snacking are frequently singled out for criticism by nutritionists and anyone passionate about maintaining a healthy lifestyle because of the dietary problems in today's environment. Notwithstanding this, moderate snacking can be a constructive way to increase your energy levels, boost your metabolism, and ensure you get enough nutrients. This dissertation will reveal ways to turn snacking from a harmful habit into a routine that benefits one's health. First, it is essential to understand the difference between nibbling because you are bored and snacking. After all, you are hungry. The first option, which is a lure promising brief pleasure, invariably results in decisions that are devoid of any nutritional value. The second option, if carried out with understanding, has the potential to maintain one's vitality throughout the day. For instance, snacks that are heavy in protein can make people feel full and stop them from overeating at following meals.

Greek yogurt, a handful of almonds, or apple slices topped with almond butter are all excellent choices for a snack. Other options include them as well. Regarding snacking sensibly, portion control appears to be a crucial component. A casual dip into a bag of chips, which could mistakenly lead to the intake of an entire day's worth of calories, can help maintain caloric balance. On the other hand, opting for pre-portioned snacks can be helpful in this regard. An individual portion of hummus and vegetables, a tiny cup of mixed vegetables, or a calibrated quantity of whole-grain crackers can serve the dual purpose of appeasing the palate and practicing the integrity of one's diet. Timing is another factor that must be taken into consideration. It is essential to ensure that snack times are determined by actual hunger rather than emotional cues for snacks to fulfill their intended purpose. The necessary fuel for the body's exercises can be supplied by eating a protein-rich snack but still relatively light an hour before physical activity.

In a similar vein, maintaining enough levels of energy and stable blood sugar can be accomplished by eating a moderate snack that is rich in nutrients between lunch and dinner. In addition, a varied snacking routine helps avoid monotonous patterns that might result in deficiencies or excesses of certain nutrients. Suppose you want to ensure your diet has many vitamins, minerals, and other essential nutrients. In that case, it is best to incorporate a wide variety of whole grains, fruits, vegetables, and nuts and seeds. This method also satisfies the taste buds by delivering a wide variety of flavors and textures that fulfill a variety of tastes. The key to successful snacking is meticulous planning and preparation. If you have access to various nutritious options, you won't feel compliant to make decisions that benefit your health. Maintaining adherence to nutritional goals is made more accessible by preparing a weekly collection of products that can be eaten as snacks, such as cut vegetables, portioned nuts, or boiled eggs. This practical method promotes both self-efficacy and the ability to withstand the allure of foods that are quick and easy to prepare. One's selection of snacks can also be improved by considering the glycemic index of the foods they eat. Foods with a lower glycemic index, such as most fruits and vegetables that are low in starch, gradually reduce glucose levels. This results in spikes in blood sugar and subsequent crashes that can lead to additional snacking. The benefits of consuming them in conjunction with a good source of fats or proteins can be appreciated.

Lastly, knowing one's physiological and psychological responses to the foods one consumes might help one make better judgments regarding snacking. Foods that make you feel sluggish or uncomfortable should be avoided, while foods that provide a consistent energy supply should be welcomed with open arms. Because people's reactions can differ significantly, it's essential to take a tailored approach to snacking.

Benefits of Homemade Snacks

Undertaking culinary advice within the confines of one's home can produce a wide variety of delicious and scrumptious snacks that are superior to those purchased from a store in terms of their level of freshness, flavor, and absence. The quest for convenience causes many people to ignore the numerous benefits of preparing snacks at home. Controlling what goes into a product is one of the most important factors because it allows individuals to accommodate individualized dietary requirements or preferences. A person's eating routine dramatically impacts their overall health, and making healthy snacks at home can be an excellent way to guarantee they are getting enough of them. These kinds of snacks often have a lower caloric count because the chef can choose ingredients that are low in sugar and do not contain high-fructose corn syrup, a common ingredient in many commercial meals. In addition, the consumption of Tran's fats, commonly found in processed foods and harmful to cardiovascular health, can be reduced or eliminated immediately from a person's diet by substituting natural fats and oils for those used in the preparation of home-cooked meals.

Additionally, homemade snacks offer a blank canvas for the incorporation of organic ingredients, which encourages a reduction in the consumption of pesticides and other chemicals that are frequently used in commercial production. When one prefers elements from organic farms or local markets, they contribute to more sustainable agricultural methods, reducing their overall environmental impact. It is indisputably true that homemade snacks are healthier than those purchased in stores because their preparation does not necessitate the use of preservatives; as a result, these snacks can be abundant in vital nutrients that are frequently stripped away during the commercial preparation process. Producing handmade snacks that satisfy the senses is another essential component of this process. The flavors are bold and can be adjusted to suit individual preferences, which pave the way for the instigation of various culinary traditions and the combination of flavors from around the world. Customizability also extends to textual aspects, one of the most critical components of a systematic portfolio. The texture of the food one consumes can be crunchy, chewy, or soft, depending on the individual's liking and the components they use. Everyone, regardless of age or skill level, can benefit tremendously from participating in the preparation of snacks because doing so provides a wealth of learning opportunities. It gives them an excellent opportunity to polish their cooking skills, understand the nutritional value of food, and cultivate a love for the art of food preparation. These kinds of activities can also foster closer links between members of the same family or group of friends, contributing to the formation of memories and customs that go beyond the mere act of providing sustenance. The manufacturing of snacks at home is frequently more viable economically. The purchase of ingredients in bulk can result in cost savings over time. This is advantageous not only for people concerned about their financial situation but also for those who want to eat food of higher quality without paying the high price tag that typically goes along with it. A more manageable budget for snacks can be maintained, and one can avoid the premiums associated with meals that have been prepared or processed. Those who suffer from food sensitivities or allergies may find that snacking on foods they have prepared for themselves positively affects their health. It is possible to verify that the atmosphere is free from cross-contamination and to carefully pick items that do not elicit allergic reactions, which offers peace of mind and makes for a safer dining experience.

Snacking for Weight Management

Snacking, which is sometimes vilified in discussions about diets that are good for your health, can, under certain conditions, contribute effectively to managing one's weight. Traditional viewpoints may criticize snacks as being unnecessary to meet daily nutritional needs; however, when incorporated into a diet strategically, they can help manage hunger and limit o during regular meals. According to conventional thinking, one must adhere to strict meal plans that leave little opportunity for additional eating if they want to manage their weight successfully. Emerging data, despite this, suggests that there may be potential benefits to including snacks as part of a diet plan, not as simple indulgencies but as components of a diet plan. This multidimensional strategy entails making a thoughtful choice of snacks, with a particular emphasis on those high in nutrients, low in caloric density, and contributing to feelings of fullness. Snacks high in fiber, such as fruits, vegetables, and whole grains, give a sense of fullness despite having a lower total calorie count. This makes it less likely that an individual will consume excessive calories. In a similar vein, eating protein-dense foods such as yogurt or almonds can keep one feeling full for longer periods, reducing the desire to eat or consume food that is not necessary. People can engage in a strategy of controlling their calorie intake without the risk of chronic hunger if they choose their options over snacks that are loaded with sugars or fats. In addition, the timing of when snacks are consumed is an important factor to consider carefully. Consuming smaller meals more frequently throughout the day can help maintain stable blood glucose levels, keep energy levels constant, and prevent the roller coaster of hunger that can commonly lead to overeating during meals. For example, eating a snack in the afternoon can prevent the outbreak of ravenous hunger that people frequently experience after work or school, leading to unhealthy eating levels. Difficulties frequently hinder efforts to regulate one's weight in terms of diet and psychological obstacles. Snacks can act as a psychological balm by offering a sense of comfort in the absence of the guilt often associated with deviating from a daily plan. They can also improve long-term dietary goals by enabling greater variety and flexibility within the diet plan. The dangers of unconscious eating, which can lead to consuming calories without awareness or enjoyment, are frequently brought up by individuals opposed to snacking. On the other hand, mindful snacking entails making decisions consciously and engaging all of one's senses while eating, which can help one develop a more harmonious connection with the food they eat. Mindful eating practices improve the quality of a snack's flavor, texture, and aroma, which promotes satisfaction with fewer portions and reduces the tendency to eat. Mindful eating practices also help reduce the risk of developing an eating disorder. Acknowledging the difference between snacking because you are hungry and eating because of your emotions is also important. Emotional eating, or comfort eating, refers to eating in response to one's emotions rather than their actual physiological hunger. To make the most of snacks as tools for weight management, it is essential to identify the signs of hunger and differentiate them from the emotional factors that cause obesity. In addition, the whole concept of a snack is going through a review now. In the past, this technique would have resulted in a packaged, processed product, but in modern times, it can result in a far larger variety of possibilities. The modern snack may be like a smoothie loaded with light grains and fruits or a tiny salad punctuated with seeds and nuts; both examples have a high nutritional density and a low caloric content. In weight control, it is necessary to frame snacks as partners rather than foes or rivals. The function of snacks in the eating process can be significantly altered by adopting a new point of view, one that sees them not as foods that derail diets but as sources of additional nutrients. This repositioning relies heavily on the recognition that practicing moderation and cautious separation is necessary. In its most basic form, snacking is a contradiction in terms. It can contribute positively to weight management, but it also has the potential to sabotage weight management efforts. Snacks, if chosen diligently and consumed with awareness, cannot only improve a person's level of dietary satisfaction but also play a pivotal role in effectively managing their weight. Snacking is currently positioned as a potential protagonist in the story of weight control, which reflects the ever-changing landscape of diet and nutrition, both constantly evolving. It urges a departure from the monolithic view of meals as the primary providers of nourishment and encourages a nuanced appreciation of eating habits. It promotes a nuanced understanding of daily habits. Snacking, if done thoughtfully and in moderation, can become an essential and beneficial device component. It is currently awaiting the incorporation of scientific knowledge and the wisdom gained from behavioral research to realize its full potential for weight control. Snacking for weight management should not be hastily disregarded or otherwise embraced without proper consideration. It requires taking a strategic approach tailored to the individual's requirements, objectives, and practices. It is a discrete variable that can be optimized, but it is neither a panacea nor a universal power. Further, it is a variable that can be maximized. Snacking can be changed from a nutritional foe into a helpful ally in maintaining a healthy weight if properly prepared and used appropriately.

Protein-Packed Snacks

Protein is a macronutrient essential for the body because it is necessary for a wide variety of processes, such as the manufacturing of enzymes and hormones and the repair and regulation of damaged tissue. High-protein snacks can be handy because they provide sustained energy, which can help maintain muscle mass, manage hunger, and promote metabolic health. Consider the lowly egg, which is a very potent source of nourishment and comes packed in its own natural shell. Eggs provide a comprehensive profile of proteins; they include all nine essential amino acids. They can be prepared in various ways, ranging from soft-boiling to poaching, making them a flexible choice for a snack. One can make them into a more complicated snack; for example, one might make devil eggs with a twist by adding avocado, which would provide a dose of beneficial fats.

Similarly, Greek yogurt is another good protein source that can be consumed. It has richer and greater consistency than its ordinary equivalent and a higher purity level than its competitor. Greek yogurt is transformed into a mouthwatering dessert when topped with a sprinkle of nuts and a drizzle of honey. The addition of the nuts not only gives the dish a satisfying crunch but also provides an increase in omega-3 fatty acids. A snack that combines chickpeas and tahini demands exploration for people with a flair for gastronomical exploration. The Middle Eastern spread known as hummus is an example of how simplicity and health can go hand in hand. It not only satisfies the palate when served with slices of cucumber or bell pepper, but it also contributes a wide variety of vitamins and minerals to the diet of everyone who consumes it.

The damaged bean holds its own when compared to other types of legumes. Both protein and fiber may be found in these young soybeans, often eaten after being cooked and lightly salted. They contribute to a feeling of fullness, preventing you from engaging in situations that aren't as good for you. Research has also been conducted on the content of these plants, which suggests that there may be potential benefits for maintaining hormone balance. A protein smoothie could benefit people who prefer sweet foods to savory foods because of the smoothie's potential sweetness. Delicious bread can be made by combining wheat or a plant-based protein powder with almond milk, frozen beans, and a dash of cinnamon. This not only gives you a boost of protein, but it also provides a wide variety of nutrients in addition to the antioxidants that come from the beans. It is important not to underestimate the practicality of nut butter, which, when spread on whole-grain toast or applied to slices, produces a sweet and satisfying snack. Consuming protein and complex carbs has been shown to maintain energy levels for longer. It's an updated take on an old favorite, and it incorporates all the nutritional know-how that contemporary dietetics has to offer. Lastly, making your protein bars at home can be fun and creative.

An easily transportable snack can be concocted by combining oats, protein powder, nut butter, and perhaps some dark chocolate chips in a small amount. These bars can be tailored to an individual's preferred flavor profile and nutritional requirements, allowing them to avoid the additives and excess sugars frequently present in their equivalents purchased from a store.

In conclusion, making high-protein snacks a regular part of one's diet can be a habit that is not only delicious but also beneficial to one's overall well-being. They are a living example of the symbiotic relationship between flavor and nutrition, proving that one does not have to compromise to get the benefits of the other. The foundation of a holistic dietary strategy is a well-rounded approach that emphasizes both diversity and moderation in food consumption. Not only does it ensure that the taste receptors are satisfied, but it also ensures that the body is nourished, maintaining both vigor and vitality.

Nutrient-Rich Vegetarian Options

In contemporary cooking, an ever-increasing emphasis has been placed on dishes that offer satisfaction without the associated guilt commonly associated with sugary confections. These desserts are not made with the typical sugar and heavy cream; they are concocted with abundant natural sweeteners, fruit purées, and innovative replacements that deliver a comparable flavor profile. In this kind of sitting, one might consider writing a dissertation about the benefits and strategies for producing these kinds of sugary delights without feeling guilty about eating them. Responses directed toward people concerned about their health have emerged due to an increased understanding of the importance of a balanced diet and the risks associated with eating sweets that are high in sugar. These tasty meals offer the body more than just filling because they contain a wide variety of components high in various nutrients, fiber, and necessary vitamins. Consider, for example, the widespread use of dates, which are a rich source of fiber and a natural source of sugar, or the incorporation of nut flours in place of refined wheat flour, which offers a plummy texture in addition to biological fats and proteins. Both of these examples are standard practices. It is possible to look at avocado chocolate mousse, a treat that combines the velvety smoothness of avocado with the deep, dark flavors of chocolate. The use of avocado, a fruit loaded with biological fats, creates a vegetarian texture comparable to that of traditional meat but does not require heavy cream or eggs. When raw cacao powder is combined with other ingredients, the end product is a delicious mousse with the appearance and texture of luxury while maintaining its high nutritional content. In addition, the function has been analyzed in great detail, which has led to the widespread use of maple syrup, honey, and even sweet spices like cinnamon and nutmeg. These natural ores provide the required while imparting the desserts with distinct flavor profiles, adding a layer of nuance. It is possible to replace processed sugar with maple syrup, which has a unique flavor and is loaded with antioxidants. This would allow social life to be maintained while simultaneously increasing health benefits. Fruit sorbet is a treat that is easy to make yet still manages to achieve sophistication, and it only requires a few essential ingredients. Sorbets, which are often made from pure fruit, a dash of lemon, and a touch of natural sugar, can satisfy a sweet tooth while still providing the nutritional advantages of the fruit used to make them. Whether it's the tangy flavor of raspberries or the subtly sweet taste of mango, sorbets are the epitome of purity and do not have any adverse effects. In addition, the use of whole grains and nuts in baking has been met with positive feedback from people concerned about their health. When almond flour or chia seeds are baked in a casserole, they add texture, flavor, essential proteins, and omega-3 fatty acids. This allows the cake or cookie to transcend its typical form.

Unsurprisingly, the culinary alchemy of baking using these substitutes can produce outcomes that are just as satisfying as their traditional analogies. The art of making s with bans and legumes is also worthy of notice because of its versatility. The ban purées of whitbans and chickpeas have been sneakily added to blondish and brownies to give these desserts a more moist consistency while increasing their protein. These concoctions shatter assumptions of what a treat may include by deftly merging the nutritious with the heavenly in a simple manner, and they are sure to blow your mind. Last but not least, any discussion about treats that don't make you feel guilty must acknowledge the contribution of dairy-free alternatives. Desserts made with coconut milk, almond milk, or soy milk provide an excellent substitute for dairy milk because they consistently maintain consistency while removing the need for lactose. When employed with the appropriate amount of forethought, these alternatives can produce ice creams and custards that can proudly take them.

Quick and Easy Snack Recipes

Without a doubt! This section contains a narrative designed to explain numerous recipes for quick and easy snacks. Amidst the frenzy of everyday chores, the search for snack concoctions that are both quick and flavorful becomes of the utmost importance. People frequently crave food that is not only nutritional but also bursting with flavor, which can be challenging to achieve when time is scarce. This practice aims to uncover dishes that combine ease of preparation with gastronomic pleasure. To begin, there is the time-honored combination of apple slices and almond butter, which one can consider. Choose an apple with a crisp, sour flavor like Granny Smith or Fuji, and cut it into tiny wedges.

Adding almond butter, full of healthy fats and proteins, makes it an ideal companion. If you gingerly dip each piece, you will have a delicious and beneficial snack. Those who prefer savory foods may find that a chickpea salad satisfies without much effort. After draining the chickpeas, combine them with chopped fresh parsley, olive oil, lemon juice, a dash of salt, and freshly cracked black pepper. Adding extra herbs or spices, such as a sprinkling of paprika or a sprinkling of Feta cheese for a Mediterranean spin, may alter this mixture. Quesadillas filled with chicken is a delicious dish that can be made with the same amount of ease as the previous one. Two tortillas, a good quantity of shredded cheese (Cheddar or Monterey Jack, your choice), and a hot pan to make one. Spread the all over one of the tortillas, cover it with the second tortilla, and then fry it in the pan until each side is golden and the inside melts into a gooey deliciousness. Eggs, which provide a blank canvas for various snack varieties, should not be undervalued because of their potential. Eggs that have been boiled can, for instance, be turned into a mouthwatering delicacy by adding a little Dijon mustard and finishing them off with a pinch of salt. Alternatively, you could make scrambled eggs and then wrap them in a warm tortilla with a sprinkle of spicy sauce to create an impromptu, delicious, and satisfying wrap. Another delicious alternative is yogurt, which is made with a variety of different ingredients.

Choose Greek yogurt instead of regular yogurt due to its velvety consistency and high protein content. Honey, granola, and fresh berries should be sprinkled on top before serving. The finished dish will have a variety of flavors and textures, including the tanginess of yogurt, the crunchiness of granola, and the sweetness of fruit and honey. It will be a symphony. One last option is to make their hummus, which is a spread that is both flexible and effortless in terms of preparation. Combine all the ingredients in a blender and process until smooth: canned chickpeas, tahini, garlic, lemon juice, and olive oil. You should experiment with other flavors and include roasted red peppers, sun-dried tomatoes, or olives in your dish. This mixture is perfect for dipping vegetables, crackers, or pita bread and tastes great on its own. Discovering that snacking does not have to be a routine or permanent act can be accomplished through these gastronomic activities. Each meal proves that it is possible to prepare food in a short amount of time that is still tantalizingly delicious and is aimed at people who want to satisfy their hunger without compromising their time. Dishes like this are a good reminder that sometimes the simplest things may be the most satisfying, particularly regarding food.

Snacking on the Go

Without a doubt, I will write an authentic, non-copyrighted essay on "Snacking on the Go" without bullet points or number rankings. The content will be close to one thousand words in length. In this day and age, where space is the distinguishing characteristic of many aspects of human effort, eating while moving around is an essential component of contemporary life. There was a time when people used to eat more quickly to keep up with the unrelenting advantage of time, but now we live in an era where the opposite is true. This evolving pattern of consumption practices involves a symphony of communication, health considerations, and cultural shifts, all of which contribute to how people indulge in transitory goods or consume their midday sustenance. Those who transport the urban sprawl seek advice in nature's vast expanses or labor in sittings that provide limited moments for respite answers to the hunger problem in today's society. Those who want to satisfy their hunger can choose from various fast food options. Choices are abundant, ranging from the unassuming cereal bar to artisanal meals loaded with various nutrients. One can choose sustenance throughout this spectrum according to their practices in terms of taste, dietary constraints, or the whims of their palate. The amount of calories and nutrients in snacks is under increasing scrutiny as people are increasingly busy and have sedentary lifestyles. Many people look for foods that might provide prolonged energy without the passive state after indulging in a fast. Options high in protein, complex carbs, and healthy fats are perfect for filling this void because they provide both satisfaction and vitality. On the other hand, alternatives high in carbohydrates and calories but don't contribute to the body's function will inevitably result in energy lows, leaving consumers exhausted and hungry for more. The social environment is also a factor in the development of snacking habits. A cornucopia of flavors has been introduced to local markets due to the branding of tastes worldwide. Consumers enjoy participating in international cuisine, as each bite provides an unspoken tale of distant locations. These kinds of snacks are not only helpful in staving off hunger but also stimulate the imagination and take the mind on a journey while simultaneously satisfying the appetite. The packaging that encloses these portable meals is of equal significance to the development of this brand. It is necessary to strike a compromise between the two goals of safeguarding the food contained and honoring sustainable agriculture's environmental imperatives. As a result, advances in materials have been made to cut down on waste without jeopardizing the safety of the food product contained within. The packaging must also provide convenience, which usually entails being simple to open, being able to be sealed again, and being robust enough to withstand the rigors of transit. It is impossible to express how beneficial to one's health it is to have snacks while traveling. The growing awareness among the general population regarding the implications of this on one's health has affected the options currently available. People often choose snacks that are not only nutritional but also curative, meaning that the substances in the snack are thought to have positive effects on both the body and the mind. These foods frequently contain vitamins, minerals, and other substances that are beneficial to one's health, which is consistent with the belief that food should serve as a substitute for medical treatments. Even though it's more convenient, nibbling on the move can often lead to unintentional consequences. For instance, the tendency to consume without attention, which frequently goes hand in hand with quick eating, might lead to obesity in certain situations. Therefore, it is still essential for consumers to take a minute, even in a hurry, to stop and think about the quantity and quality of what they are consuming. Technology has also played a part in developing portable devices in recent years. Individuals can now keep track of their consumption, understand the nutritional composition of the snacks they eat, and make informed decisions based on the daily activities they have set for themselves, thanks to applications for smartphones and other devices. This intersection of technology and data provides a sense of control, countering the discomfort of living a fast-paced life. In addition, the social aspect of snacking should not be overshadowed by the individualistic characteristics of a snack consumed in a hurry. An act of camaraderie, a moment of communion with other people, or just an excuse for social engagement can all be accomplished by sharing a snack. Snacks are frequently the pivot around which talks revolve, which in turn helps to strengthen connections. It is necessary to educate people on the implications of their food choices, particularly when such choices are made quickly. Consumers are helped to navigate the myriad choices available to them by programs and campaigns that provide information about the nutritional worth of various snacks as well as the potential health consequences that those snacks may have. Regarding eating habits, these educational campaigns frequently promote moderation, diversity, and a sense of balance. It would appear that advancements in food science, shifts in cultural behaviors, and innovations in packaging and technology will all play a role in the future of eating while on the move. New nutritional front liners may offer foods that

Snacks for Energy and Focus

Maintaining one's productivity throughout the day requires a significant amount of both energy and focus. As a result of the fact that continuous lifestyles frequently require constant attention and vigor from individuals, making intelligent snack choices is not simply an issue of sustaining cognitive and physical performance but also of ensuring that one is not hungry. It has been demonstrated that consuming foods high in complex carbs, proteins, and healthy fats effectively provides sustainable energy and improves nutrition. This discussion will shed light on the qualities of such snacks and their function in enhancing one's ability to concentrate and maintain energy levels. It is impossible to discount the role of nuts in terms of their ability to improve mental and physical performance. For example, almonds contain a wealth of biological fats, proteins, and magnesium, a well-known mineral for its contribution to generating energy at the cell level. A moderate amount can make you feel hungry while boosting the body's energy stores. Thanks to the amount of omega-3 fatty acids they contain, walnuts also contribute to the health of cerebral tissue and, consequently, to the clarity of cognitive function. Oatmeal is an excellent choice for breakfast because it has a low glycemic index, which allows for a more controlled delivery of glucose into the bloodstream than other morning foods. This steady release of energy helps prevent the dramatic spikes and troughs in blood sugar levels that are frequently blamed for the energy slumps that occur in the Middle of the morning. Sustenance, such as that required for sustained attention, can be provided by a bowl of oats, which the addition of some butter or a dab of nut butter might improve. Greek yogurt is another worthy choice to help you maintain energy throughout the day. The moderate amount of sugar combined with the substantial amount of protein helps the body gradually release its stored energy. In addition, the practice of probiotics is beneficial to gut health, which, through an axis known as the gut-brain connection, is surprisingly linked to cognitive health. Eggs, frequently referred to as nature's multivitamin, include all of the essential amino acids and a variety of nutrients, such as choline, which is vital for maintaining healthy brain function. Eating a hard-boiled egg, whether as a solitary snack or as part of a more substantial meal, makes a major contribution to this combination; it satisfies one's hunger and ensures a constant energy source. The natural sugars in the fruit provide an immediate rush of energy, but the fruit's fiber ensures slow and continuous absorption.

The fat and protein in the pumpkin butter also help maintain energy levels. Dark chocolate is a perfect buddy to have on hand for those times when the focus is flagging, and a quick pick-me-up is required. The flavones found in cacao have been linked to improved cognitive performance, and the small amount of caffeine it contains delivers an immediate boost in focus, although that is only temporary. Pumpkin seeds are a snack that isn't as well-known but is effective for boosting concentration and energy. Antioxidants, magnesium, zinc, and fatty acids are all essential for maintaining a healthy brain, and these substances are a treasure trove of these crucial nutrients.

In conclusion, the many advantages of staying well-hydrated must not be overlooked. Learning symptoms and a reduction in cognitive function can be brought on by dehydration. There is some evidence that drinking herbal teas, particularly ones infused with ginseng or ginkgo balboa can improve mental health and performance. When these beverages are eaten instead of those heavy in sugar, they deliver hydration without the unfavorable effects associated with sugar crashes. Keeping one's energy and concentration levels up throughout the day is complex and uniquely individual. However, including some of the snacks listed above in your diet can significantly benefit both sustained cognitive and physical performance. Thanks to the one-of-a-kind combination of nutrients, every snack satisfies the body's complex requirements for energy and helps the mind stay focused. It is in the best interest of individuals to consider their snack choices not just as transitory moments of enjoyment but as essential components of a lifestyle structured for optimal performance and mental clarity.

Allergen-Friendly Snacking

Eating in a way that is safe for people who have food allergies has become of the utmost significance in our day and age, when daily limitations are not only personal practices but vital health regulations for many people. It is an issue that merits discussion and serious investigation to ensure that nutritional options are accessible to everyone. Snacks, one of the most common allergens, offer more than sustenance. Those burdened by the restrictions of their daily lives can look to them as a guiding light toward normalcy. Individuals with food sensitivities can participate in the communal feast thanks to the provision of these edible offerings, which eliminates the risk of an allergic reaction. As a result, the supply of such snacks is not just a sign of civility but also a significant act of empathy on the part of the host. Throughout history, snacking has been treated as a casual activity, rarely given the appropriate thought it deserves, particularly regarding its potential to induce undeniable consequences.

However, there has been a change brought about by modernity. As a result of the frequency of allopathic disorders, a sizable portion of the population must now carefully examine each bite they take. This problem is made much more difficult by the widespread allergens in normal snack foods, such as peanuts, grains, dairy products, soy, eggs, and shellfish. Making snacks that are safe for people with allergies requires careful consideration when choosing the components and awareness of the potential for cross-contamination. To ensure no allergic proteins are present, each component needs to be thoroughly examined, and its provision needs to be confirmed. In addition, producers are required to control painstakingly and, if not eliminate, at least minimize their employees' exposure to the various hazards present in the workplace. These snacks are appealing not just because they are risk-free but also because of the high quality of the food they contain and how tasty they are. They have to perform the dual job of nourishing the body while appetizing the taste buds. To accomplish this goal, innovative culinary experiences and advancements in food technology must come together. For example, almond milk has gained popularity as an alternative to traditional dairy products, and coconut flour can be used as a suitable replacement for traditional wheat flour. A look at the available products today reveals an expanding selection of snacks that do not contain common allergens. Fruits, inherently devoid of these reactive proteins, have emerged as an essential component in this industry. Delicious delicacies can also be crafted from vegetables using preparation techniques such as drying, baking, or roasting. These are not mere substitutes; they are stand-alone devices that a diverse group of people enjoy. The prevalence of soy and nuts in foods rich in protein makes it difficult to create snacks safe for people with allergies to these foods. Protein is an essential nutrient. These seeds may frequently be obtained as desirable alternatives, roasted as snacks, or included in bars. Another source is legumes, except peanuts; chickpeas, in particular, are typically baked into a crunchy and savory snack. In this context, flavor's fundamental role is not something that can be ignored. To produce the desired flavor without introducing ingredients, careful use of seasonings and spices is required during cooking. As a result, flavoring becomes an exercise in culinary skills in which one seeks to balance flavor and digestive safety. Despite these developments, there are still barriers to the process of developing snacks that are safe for those with allergies. The cost is a significant consideration since the acquisition of specialist industries and the upkeep of production lines from all sides can increase costs. These costs are then passed on to the user, raising concerns about the product's affordability. Despite this, one could reasonably predict that economies of scale will ultimately reduce the security of their financial assets as the level of demand continues to rise. A fair strategy for snacking requirements requires, in addition, careful attention to the clarity of product labeling. The specific state of common laws on product packaging is now required by law in several jurisdictions worldwide. This transparency is essential because it allows individuals to make well-informed choices regarding the consumables they purchase. The case for safe snacks for those with food allergies is strengthened when it is considered in the context of educational institutions. Young students, particularly those still in the elementary grades, may not have the discipline required to stay away from all Snacks that are safe for those with food allergies, symbolic of a larger cultural change toward greater diversity in daily choices. They reflect a rising acknowledgment of the diversity of human physiology and the accompanying variety of requirements that go along with it. As time goes on and more people become aware of and educated about food allergies, it is quite likely that this pattern will remain consistent. The culinary environment is continuously changing, with establishments constantly adapting their offerings to meet the complex requirements of an increasingly diverse clientele. Snacks that do not include all ingredients are at the forefront of this revolution; they symbolize a future in which everyone can enjoy food without fear, without taking any risks, and with great joy.

Special Diet Snacks (Kato, Pale)

When delving into the nuance of gastronomic tastes consistent with specialist nutritional regimes such as the Neolithic and Paleolithic diets, it is necessary to acknowledge the fundamental differences between these eating styles and more traditional approaches to food preparation. People who follow these rules frequently look for snack options that are accessible according to the regulation's tight guidelines. In this section, we will discuss a variety of tasty snacks that are appropriate for various diets. We will also explain how these snacks can be prepared and their nutritional profiles. Or "Kato" snacks have a composition that is high in fat, has a moderate amount of protein, and has a low amount of carbohydrates. They have to satiate their hunger while keeping their metabolism in a state known as ketosis, in which the body burns fat rather than glucose for energy.

On the other hand, snacks that adhere to the Paleolithic, or "Palo," avoid processed foods, wheat, and dairy products in favor of foods said to have been consumed during the Paleolithic period. Crisps are a delicious and practical alternative for those who follow the diet. One can make a snack high in fat and flavor by baking pieces of shredded cheese until they attain a golden crisp. This results in the creation of a snack. The avocado, a fruit with emollient characteristics, makes for a good snack when consumed on its own or in conjunction with other components, such as guacamole, which is finished with vegetables rather than corn chips. Both the diet and the pale diet rely heavily on nuts and seeds as a source of the heart-healthy lipids they contain. Raw or lightly roasted almonds, macadamias, and walnuts seasoned with unrefined sea salt are the most popular preparations for these nuts.

Due to the high caloric density of these foods, modifications in their consumption are required, particularly when following a k diet, which places a premium on maintaining a healthy balance of macronutrients. Moving on to the pale sector, we discovered that fresh vegetables accompanied by a handmade dip, such as nut butter or a sauce based on tahini, are in perfect accordance with the day's flavors. The crunch's basis lies within the domain of what would be available in a culture of hunters and gatherers, which is the primary focus of this discussion, along with the snack's minimally processed character. Jerky, another option for a snack, has seen a surge in popularity, particularly grass-fed types free of artificial preservatives and additional sugars. This source of protein is particularly suitable for ingestion while on the move, which is a blessing for the contemporary Homo sapiens, who are also concerned about their health. When it comes to fruit, those following the Pale diet might opt for berries or slices of melon because these types of fruit have lower sugar and a higher nutritional content than other fruits. Within the scope of a dish that is often high in savory and umami flavors, its inherent sweetness might function as a reward. Those who are following a diet, on the other hand, need to be very careful about how much fruit they eat because the fructose in fruit might throw off ketosis. The coconut milk smoothie is a culinary concoction loved by people adhering to both paled diets. One can make a satiating mix that is refreshing and rich in nutrients by blending full-fat coconut milk with a small portion of broccoli and possibly a handful of spinach. This will produce the desired results. In addition, eggs that have been hard-boiled provide an excellent snack that is compatible with each other. They deliver a variety of vitamins and are loaded with high-quality proteins, lipids, and other essential nutrients. It is possible to improve these foods' flavor and nutritional value by seasoning them with spices such as smoky paprika and turmeric. When coming up with snacks to accompany these diets, one must never forget the overall daily impression and how a particular snack fits into the broader framework of the diet. It is not just an issue of what is allowed but also of what is beneficial for maintaining the nutritional equilibrium necessary for these diets.

To summarize, although the restrictions imposed by the diets may, at first glance, give the impression that they restrict the variety of snacks that may be consumed, in reality, they encourage innovation in the diet. They promote eating whole foods rich in nutrients, which can transform snacking from a simple act of delight into a show that nourishes the body. These diets, when adhered to with diligence and forethought, can bring tremendous benefits, transforming not only the metabolism of the body but also the relationship an individual has with the food they eat.

Mindful Snacking and Portion Control

The key to maintaining a healthy, well-balanced diet and ensuring that a person's dietary intake is consistent with their physiological requirements is to practice mindful snacking and to keep portion sizes under control. This book aims to shed light on the value of mindful snacking, various tactics for controlling portion sizes, and the attendant advantages that result from such activities. Snacking, frequently misconstrued as little more than an indulgence, can serve a biological purpose. When practiced with awareness, it can satisfy hunger between meals, maintain a healthy blood sugar level, and give you energy. A snack involves paying attention not just to the signs that the body is sending but also to the food's nutritional content. This action goes beyond simply consuming food and develops into cultivating awareness of oneself and caring for oneself. The compulsory practice of controlling one's portion sizes requires exercising discretion about the amount of food one eats. This helps to ensure that the caloric and nutritional requirements of the body are met without fail. Before one can snack thoughtfully, one must identify the factors that cause them to want to munch on something between meals. Emotional states such as stress or boredom, indications from the surrounding environment, or even actual hunger could be among the potential triggers. The distinction between these catalysts is of the utmost importance. As soon as the motivation is understood, food choice becomes extremely important. Options higher in fiber, protein, and healthy fats are frequently advised in place of options high in refined carbohydrates and contain no nutritional value whatsoever. Choices such as a piece of fruit, a handful of almonds, or a portion of Greek yogurt contribute to feelings of fullness and provide adequate nutrients. Consequentially, the capacity of an individual to determine the proper quantity of food necessary to satisfy hunger without leading to overeating is an essential component of effective portion management. Utilizing smaller plates for meals, portioning snacks into single-serving containers, and avoiding eating food directly from the packaging are some strategies that can be used to accomplish this objective. Eating slowly establishes the body's signals of satisfaction to reach the brain, which promotes a sense of fullness despite consuming less food. This makes it easier to exercise moderation in eating, which can also be assisted by eating slowly. The combination of mindful snacking and portion control brings with it a multitude of potential benefits. This dynamic duo may play an essential part in modifying caloric intake for people who want to maintain their weight while still maintaining their ability to enjoy their favorite foods. In addition, these practices promote a harmonious relationship with food, in which the individual no longer consumes for the only purpose of pleasure or out of compulsion but rather to nourish themselves and improve their health. Additional benefits commonly associated with this method include increased levels of energy, improved digestive health, and a strengthened immune system. A scholarly examination of this subject suggests that mindful eating practices, such as snacking with intention and regulating portion sizes, may also benefit mental health. The self-discipline required to adhere to such routines can instill practitioners with a stronger sense of control over their lives, which can contribute to an improvement in mood and an anxiety reduction caused by concerns about one's body image and the food choices one makes.

Furthermore, it is essential to recognize that this path is highly individualized, and what is beneficial to one person may not be appropriate for another. Several factors, including cultural norms, physiological conditions, and personal preferences, can significantly influence an individual's approach to snacking and portion sizes. Therefore, the ability to be flexible and adaptable is essential.

Snacking for Special Occasions

A significant part of the celebrations customarily associated with special events is consuming various disposable foods, including snacks. These durable materials, which have been meticulously picked and manufactured, satisfy the attendees' taste buds and contribute to the general atmosphere and the environment. The purpose of this presentation is to illustrate the art of selecting and making snacks appropriate for various celebrations and events. It is essential to reach a consensus that snacks are not only a filler between meals but an outlet for the experience of one's creativity in the kitchen. They have the potential to break the ice, make it easier for attendees to mix, and keep everyone entertained. When dealing with the problem of selecting suitable snacks, one must consider the event's nature, the attendees' gustatory preferences, and the smooth integration of the snacks into the overall narrative of the gourmet experience. For example, for a wedding reception, the joining of two lives is a momentous occasion, and the reactions during the reception should reflect the occasion's significance. As a result, the options might include dainty canapés, bite-sized bruschetta topped with a variety of sophisticated toppings, and petite fours that emit an air of refined refinement. Each nibble not only provides food but also acts as an invitation to the joyous occasion that is being celebrated. When holidays like the Lunar New Year or Diwali are imbued with cultural importance, such as when they are observed, snacks become a means through which traditions are preserved and shared. It is possible to find lads and spring rolls there. Spring rolls are associated with riches because of their similarity to gold bars, and Ladinos are supposed to bring good fortune. These bite-sized morsels are steeped in a rich cultural history and perfectly capture the occasion's spirit perfectly.

On the other hand, substantial and hearty snacks are often appropriate for less formal get-togethers, such as gaming events or casual get-togethers with friends. Customers typically go for dishes like loaded nachos, hot wings, or sliders when given the choice. They are items that can be consumed and contribute to the laid-back and hearty ambiance typically maintained at the end of this year. When preparing snacks for special events, the separation is not the only thing that matters; the practice is also. Visual appeal is of the utmost importance; a skillfully prepared snack can both whet the hunger and soothe as a topic of conversation. Therefore, paying careful attention to the particulars, such as the selection of serving plates and garnishing, becomes just as essential as understanding the flavor profile. In addition to that, diary concerns are necessary. In this day and age, when food allegiances, intolerances, and dietary practices are mo. This will guarantee that everyone feels welcome. This kind of attention to detail in catering contributes to all guests' overall comfort and satisfaction. Timing is of the utmost importance when it comes to the creation of these delivery targets. Snacks typically satisfy hunger without interfering with one's ability to enjoy the main dish. As a result, the dimensions of these snacks have been adjusted so that they are sufficiently filling without being excessively so. An additional feature worthy of attention is the provision of resources as intangibles during events with effective processes. Snacks, for example, might serve as a nice break during long events like conferences or seminars, allowing attendees' minds to relax and rest. One might find bite-sized versions of quiches, skewers of mixed fruits, or energy balls, all offering food without bringing on feelings of lethargic drowsiness.

www.ingramcontent.com/pod-product-compliance
Lightning Source LLC
Chambersburg PA
CBHW070733260726
48660CB00007B/2819